I0703192

NOURISH YOU

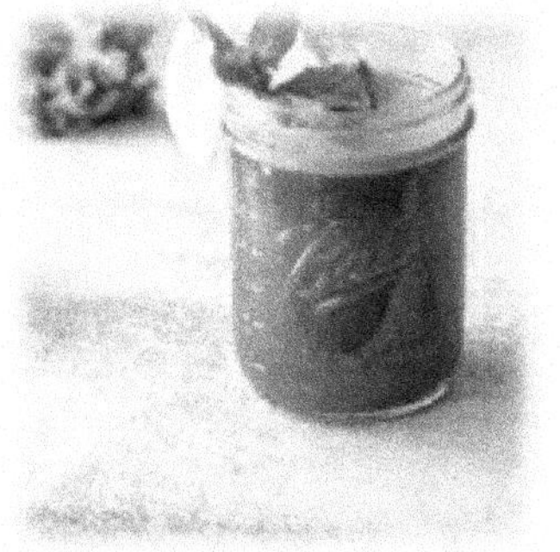

María Casado Cuyás

5

Introduction
WHAT IS WELLNESS

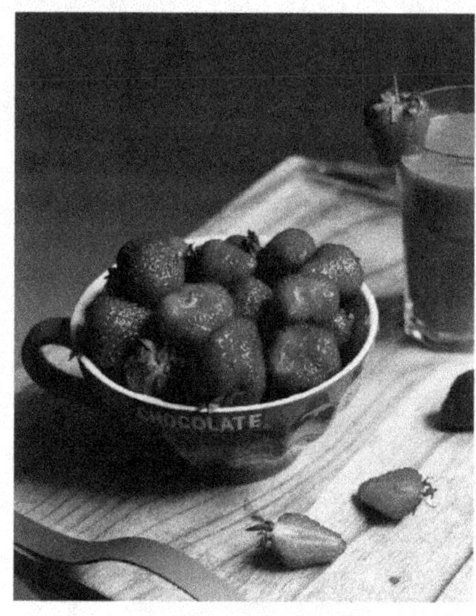

YOU ARE
WHAT YOU EAT

You reflect outside what you put into your body, through the nourishment you give yourself, not only with food but also with your thoughts

BREAKFAST

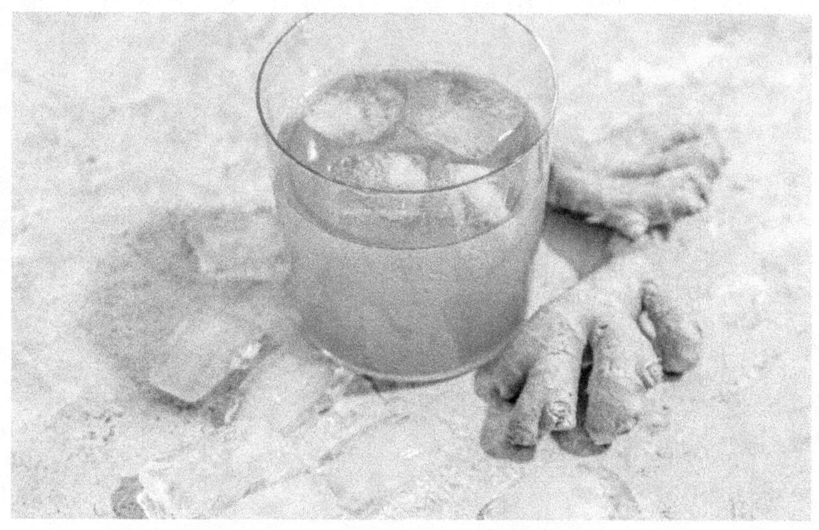

I enclose here my favourite

recipes

New Earth   @mariakrystalflames

Breakfast

PLAN YOUR MEALS

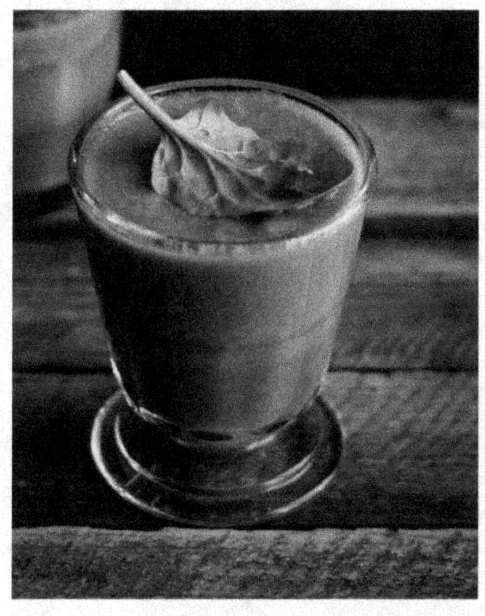

Detox

Take care of you

eat healthy food snacks

Get 7 hours of sleep

Enjoy stillness and

meditate

Spend time in nature

New Earth   @mariakrystalflames

RECIPES

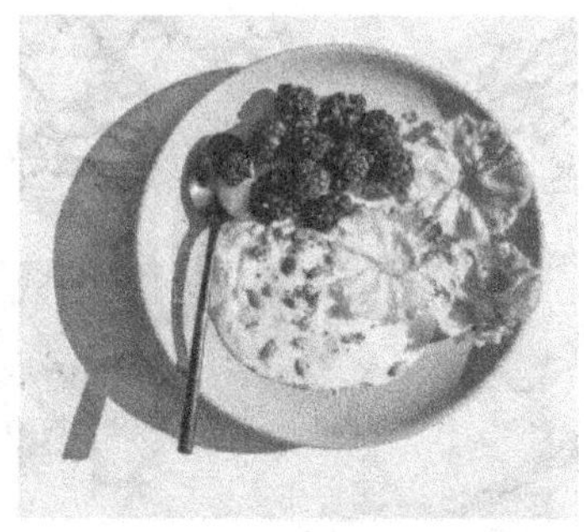

BOWL WITH FRUITS

Ingredients

- 1l liquid yogurt
- Assorted fruits
- honey
- nuts
- seeds

Preparation

Just pour in the liquid yogurt and garnish it with fruits to your liking, some nuts and honey.

RECIPES

Ingredients

- 4 tablespoons rolled oats
- fresh fruits
- 500 ml water or veggie drink
- 3 nuts and raisins
- cinnamon, honey or salt

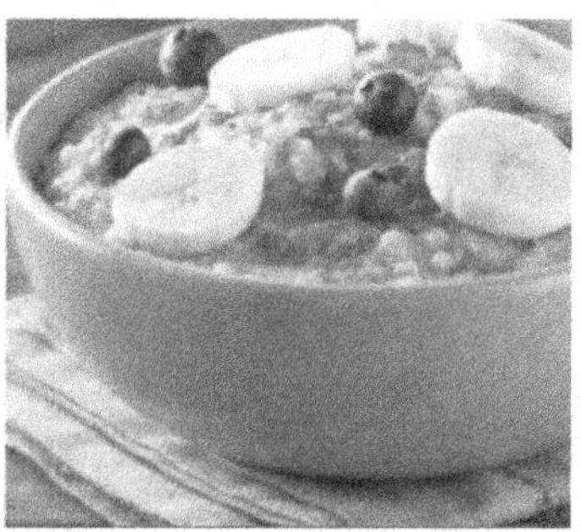

PORRIDGE

Preparation

Porridge, is very popular due to its laxative effects, it is healthy & nutritious Put the water on the heat, when it bubbles to boil add the oat flakes. After 10 minutes they are ready.

You can consume it when it cools down by adding fruit and nuts or some yogurt to your liking. I leave it prepared the night before in the fridge. So, the next morning I only have to serve myself breakfast.

RECIPES

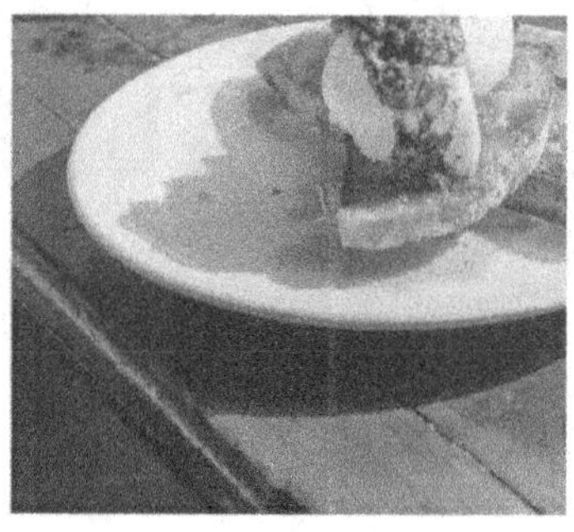

WHOLE WHEAT
TOAST

Ingredients

- rustic bread
- vegan cheese
- oil
- a couple of cloves of garlic
- fresh parsley

Preparation

Cut the bread into slices and toast it
Brush it with the garlic clove.
Mix and mash another clove of garlic
with fresh parsley and oil
Place the mash on the toast.
You can accompany it with nuts and
honey

RECIPES

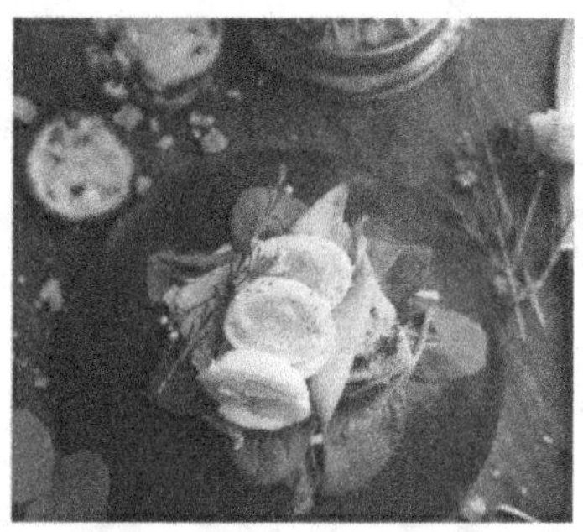

AVOCADO TOAST

Ingredients

- Wholemeal bread
- Avocado and cheese
- Oil and garlic
- A couple of eggs

Preparation

Cut the bread into slices and toast it
Brush it with the garlic clove and
drizzle it with oil
Put the egg to cook for 9 minutes or 7
if you prefer it poached
You can accompany it with raisins,
walnuts and honey
Ready to serve

14

AT NOON

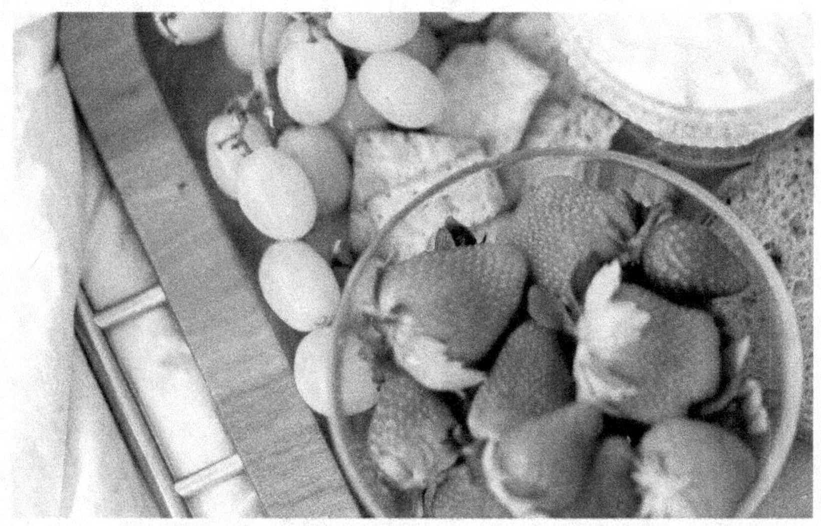

I enclose here some appetizers

New Earth   @mariakrystalflames

Snacks
AT NOON

Eat healthy snacks

a fruits bowl

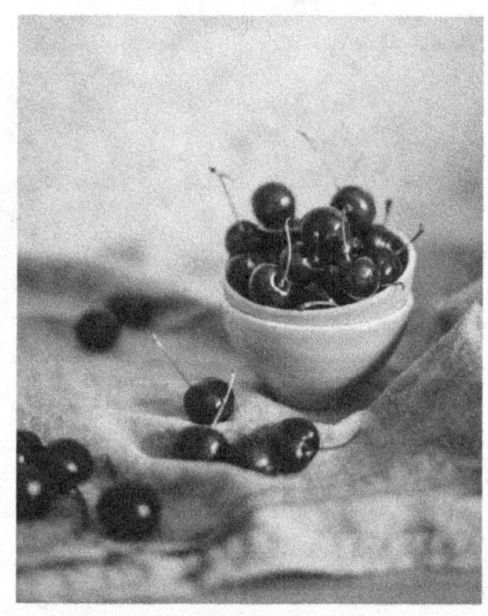

RECIPES

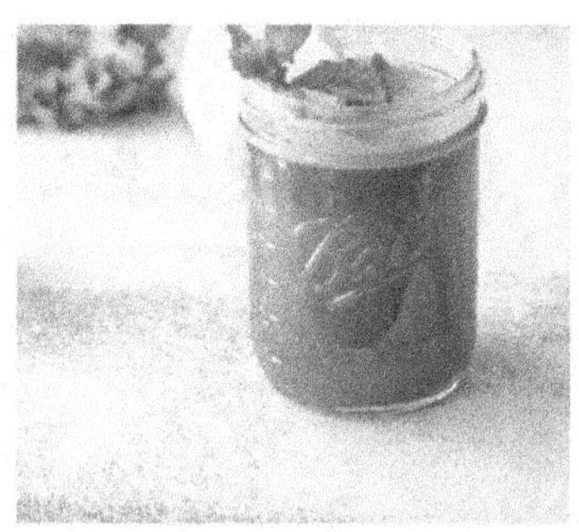

SPINACH SMOOTHIE

Ingredients

- spinachs
- a banana
- oat milk
- honey (optional)

Preparation

Wash the spinach and cut the banana into slices. Place everything in the blender with water or plant-based milk and a little honey and cinnamon.

Keep what you don't consume on the go in the fridge

RECIPES

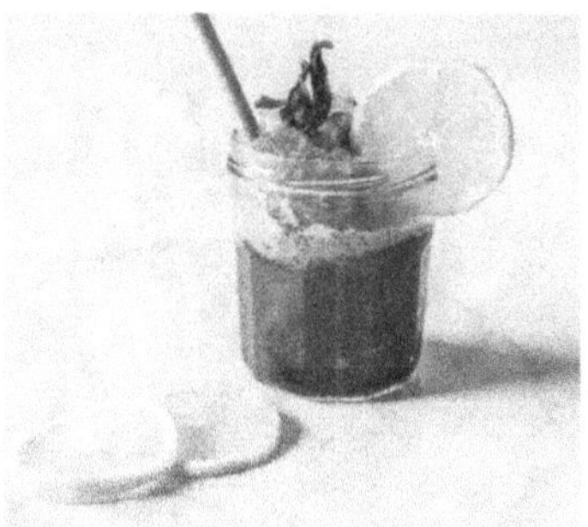

BEETROOT SMOOTHIE

Ingredients

- beetroot
- a banana
- 2 glasses of water

Preparation

Cut the banana & the beetroot into slices. Place everything in the blender with water or plant-based milk.

Keep what you don't consume on the go in the fridge

RECIPES

Ingredients

- 1/2 vegetable milk
- 1 teaspoon ground turmeric
- 1 piece of fresh ginger
- Cinnamon and pepper

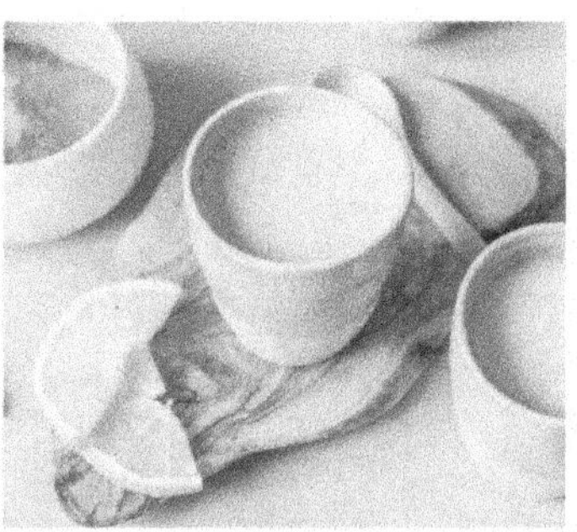

GOLDEN MILK

Preparation

Heat the plant-based milk in a small saucepan, stir and add the rest of the ingredients: turmeric, grated ginger, cinnamon, pepper and honey to taste.

Remember to drink plenty of water or refreshing infusions

LUNCHS

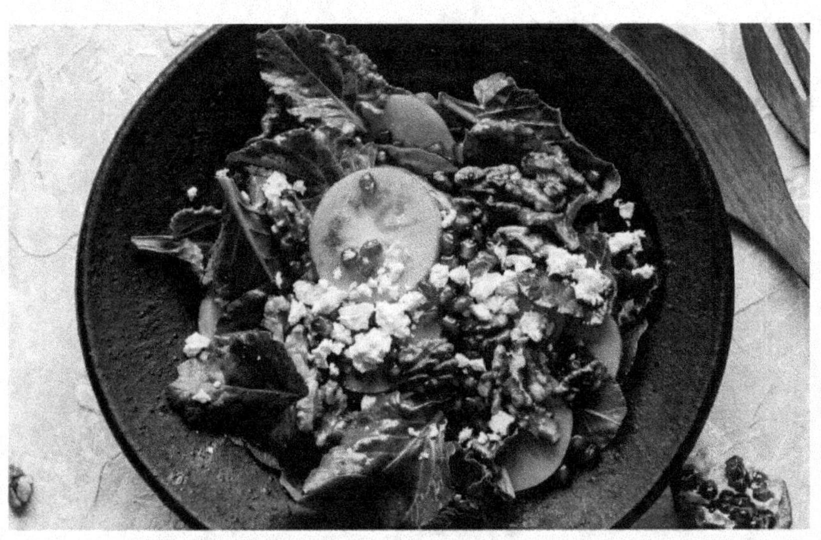

HEALTHY

New Earth   @mariakrystalflames

Lunch

PLAN AHEAD

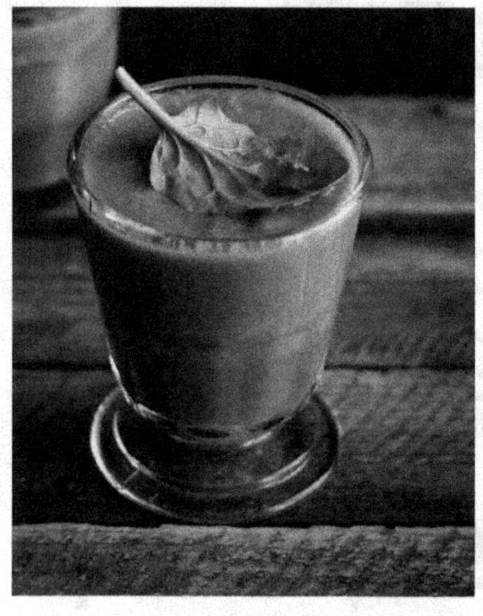

Replenish

I enclose my best recipes for a good nourishment

New Earth   @mariakrystalflames

RECIPES

Ingredients

- 250grs watercress & pinto beans
- 2 potatoes
- 250grs pumpkin and carrot
- 2 corn cones cut in half

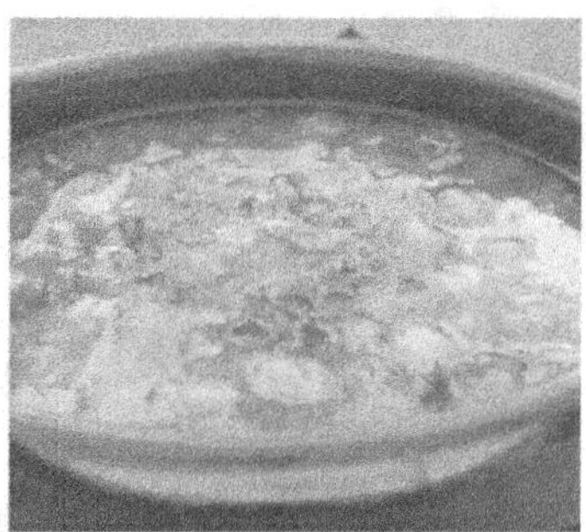

WATERCRESS SOUP

Preparation

The day before, we let the beans soak.
The next day, we start with the onion and garlic stir-fry.
While they are browning, we are preparing the rest of the ingredients, chopping the watercress into pieces, peeling and dicing the pumpkin, carrot and potatoes

Once the onion is poached, with the carrot and pumpkin.
Prepare the potatoes, some corncones, watercress in a cauldron, adding the poached onion with carrot & pumpkin and covering everything with water. If you use a pressure cooker, it will be ready in 45 minutes

RECIPES

Ingredients

- 2 leeks, 1 carrot and zucchini
- 1 cup spinach leaves
- 2 cups evaporated milk
- 2 tablespoons olive oil

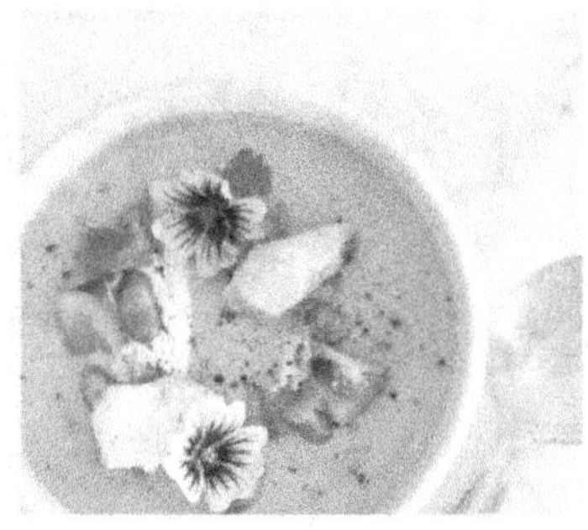

VEGGIE CREAM

Preparation

Well washed, the leeks are cut into slices and the zucchini and carrot into small squares.
Then, over low heat, fry in oil until they begin to brown.
Put the spinach to boil for 10 minutes.
Then, if you want to thicken, pour in the evaporated milk or cornmeal until you get a fine cream. Season with salt and pepper to taste.

RECIPES

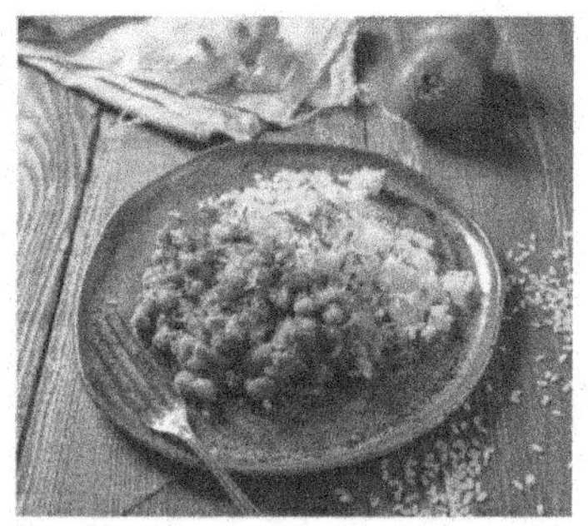

RICE WITH CHICKPEAS

Ingredients

- 1 head of garlic, a tomato
- 1/2 red or green pepper
- 400 grs. of rice
- 1/2 grs. of chickpeas

Preparation

Sauté the garlic with the peppers and tomato while boiling the rice. Lately for convenience I already use chickpeas prepared in a glass jar. But you can also cook them in a pressure cooker after soaking them the night before with a little baking soda to soften them.

Place all the ingredients in a pan and put them on the heat for a few more minutes so that the flavours merge.

RECIPES

Ingredients

- 500grs chickpeas & a cabbage
- 4 potatoes, 3 carrots and 1 leek
- 100 grs thin noodles
- olive oil and salt

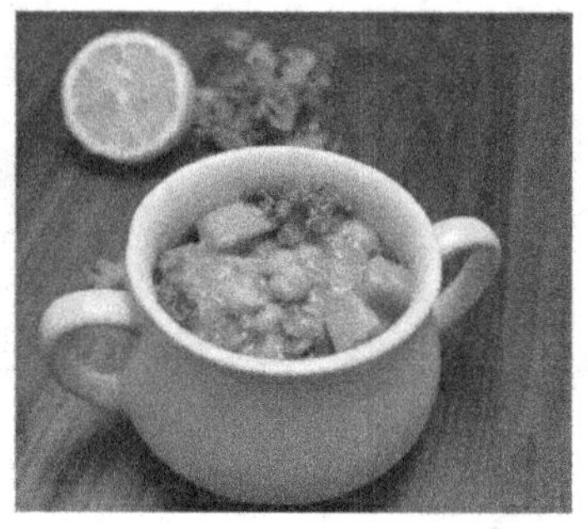

VEGETARIAN
CHICKPEAS STEW

Preparation

Soak the chickpeas the night before.
In a clay pot place the chickpeas and vegetables,
Cook everything for 30 minutes in the oven. Or in a normal casserole and then present it in the clay casserole.
Once everything is finished cooking, remove the broth for the soup
To make the soup, strain the broth and add the noodles to boil. The cooking time of the thin noodle is around 7 min

RECIPES

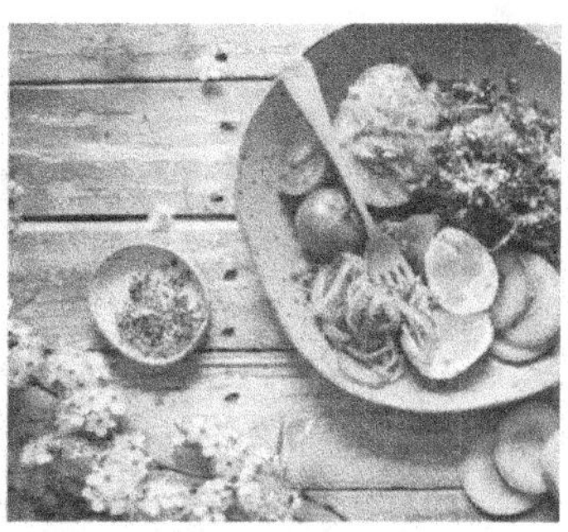

TENDER SPROUT
SALAD

Ingredients

- lettuce & spinach in tender sprouts

- onion & feta cheese

- oil, vinegar and honey

- nuts and raisins

Preparation

Just mix the ingredients well in a bowl
and you will have them ready to serve.

It is an ideal choice for spring

RECIPES

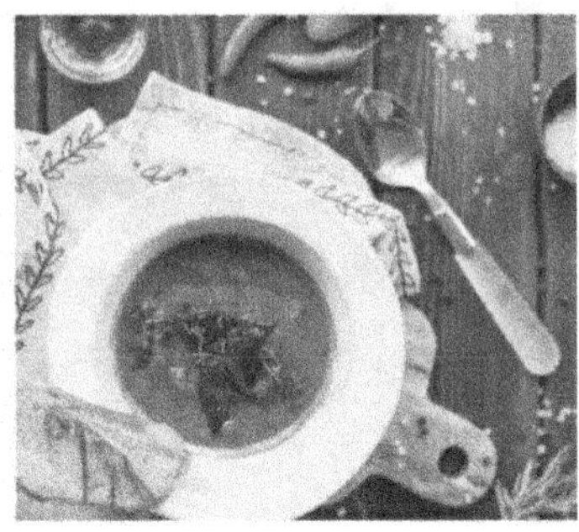

GAZPACHO

Ingredients

- 3 tomatoes, an onion, a cucumber
- a green pepper
- 30 grs of bread crumbs
- vinegar, oil and salt

Preparation

Wash the tomatoes and green peppers, chop them and put them in the blender glass.

Also chop the spring onion, garlic clove and cucumber and add everything to the jug. Chop the breadcrumbs and add it. Season, pour a splash of vinegar and a good splash of olive oil.
Blend all the ingredients with the blender and serve them in a jar

RECIPES

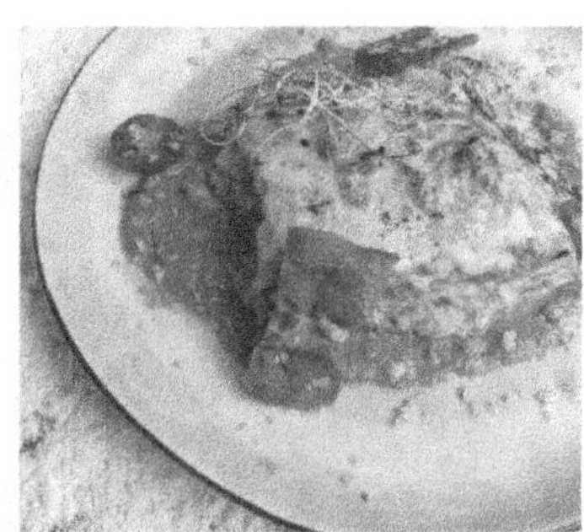

SPINACH LASAGNA

Ingredients

- Lasagna pasta sheets
- 250 grs spinachs
- fluor, butter, vegan milk
- oil, cheese, onion & garlic

Preparation

Boil the pasta sheets and remove them to a plate of cold water.
Sauté the flour with the butter while stirring until it begins to brown; Add the vegan milk a little at a time while mixing. Once all the milk is integrated, add the cheese and salt and pepper

Sauté the spinach with the onion and garlic in a frying pan over medium heat with the olive oil. On a tray, place a layer of pasta and a thin layer of spinach. Repeat this three times and finish with the béchamel sauce.
Sprinkle the Parmesan cheese over the lasagna and bake at 175° C for 40 minutes.

RECIPES

Ingredients

- 180 grs tagliatelle pasta
- 200 grs spinachs
- an onion & garlic
- 175 ml. of cooking cream

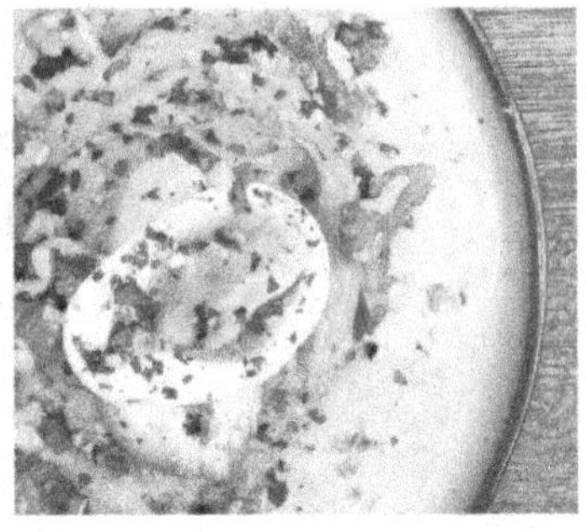

TAGLIATELLE PASTA
WITH SPINACHS

Preparation

Cook the pasta for 7 minutes in the cauldron
Sauté the onion with the spinach and mushrooms.
When they are fried, add the cream and let it rest in the pan for a few minutes to thicken the cream.
Serve on a plate and sprinkle with cheese on top
We can add raisins, pine nuts or olives to taste

Snacks
FOR THE EVENING

Nourish yourself
eat healthy snacks

a fruits bowl

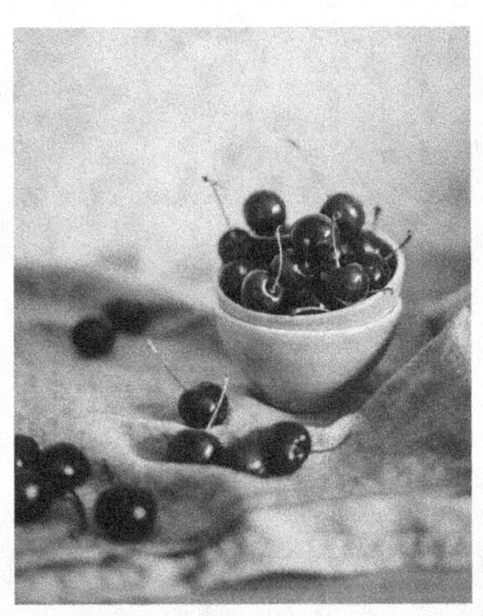

New Earth   @mariakrystalflames

APPETIZERS

avocado toast

olives & cheese

smoothies

healthy snacks

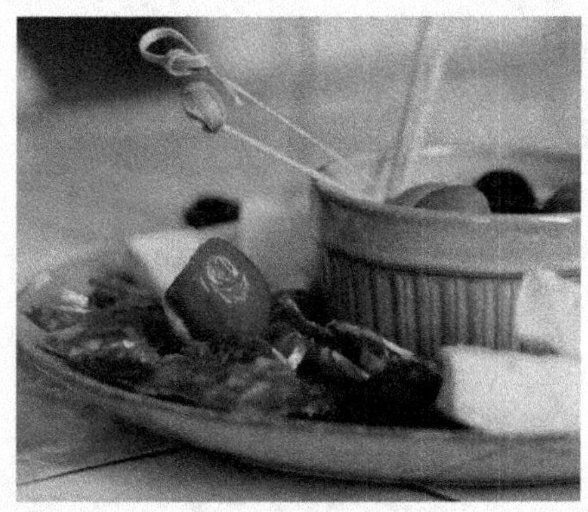

DINERS

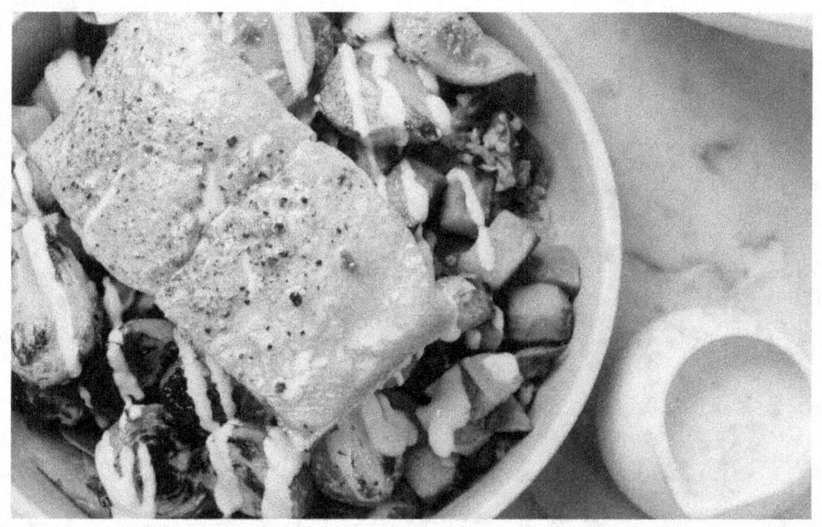

I enclose here my healthy

favourites recipes

New Earth   @mariakrystalflames

Diner
PLAN YOUR DINERS

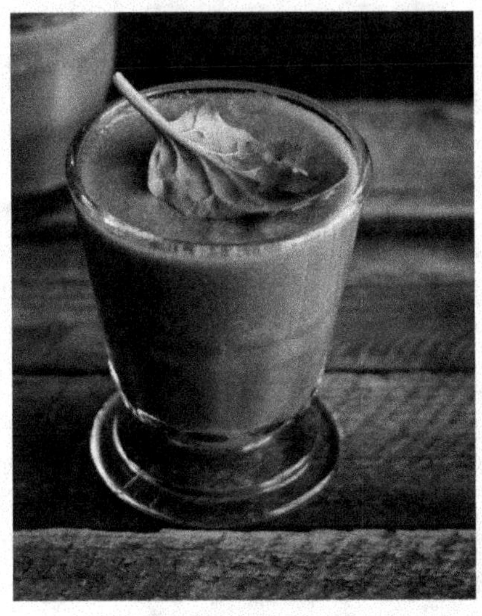

Prepare your body to
sleep with a gentle
super

Take care

RECIPES

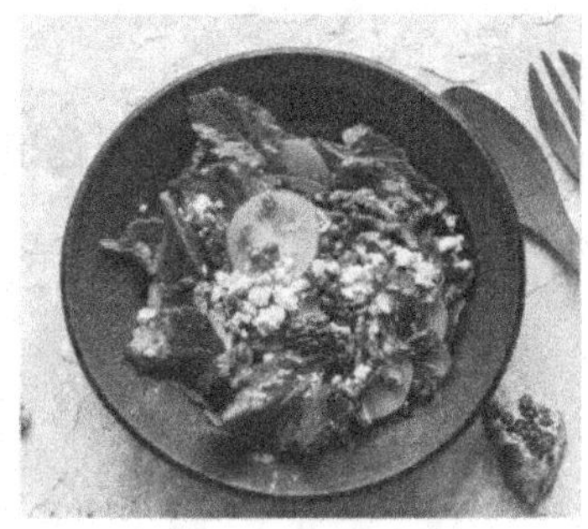

SAUTÉED SPINACHS

Ingredients

- 250 grs spinachs
- Pine nuts to taste
- 2 cloves of garlic
- Oil and salt

Preparation

In a frying pan with a little oil on the bottom, fry the garlic until golden brown. Reserve.

In the same pan, fry the pine nuts until golden brown and take them out on a separate plate with the garlic.

Put the spinach in the pan and turn it for about 10 minutes over medium heat, so that the water they keep releasing evaporates.

Just before removing from the heat, add the garlic and pine nuts and mix.

RECIPES

Ingredients

5 leeks and 2 potatoes

50 grs. butter

850 ml. of broth

200 ml. of cream

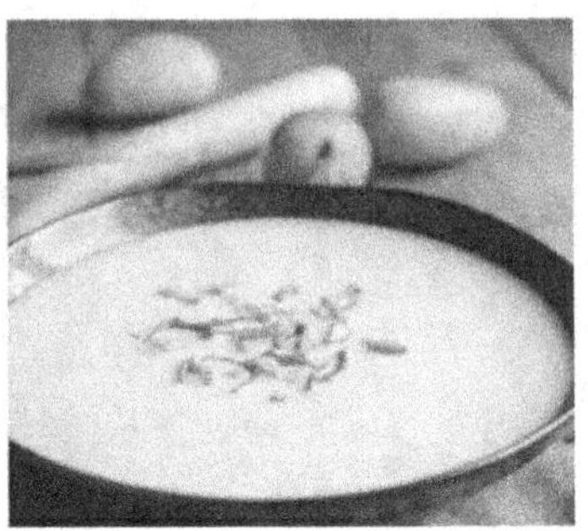

VICHYSSOISE

Preparation

To prepare the recipe for vichyssoise or cream of leeks we are going to use only the white part of these vegetables, so we cut the white part of the leek and remove the outermost layer.
Wash them well and cut into thin slices.
Peel, wash and chop the potatoes.
Now, in a saucepan, put the butter to heat over low heat. Add the leek and let it cook

Add the pieces of potato and pour all the broth on top. At this point increase the heat a little and let everything cook together for about 25 minutes.
Beat it with the blender. Pour in the cream and mix everything together. Store it in the fridge until it's time to serve it.
You can prepare a variant with zucchini, carrot or pumpkin cream, in which case you may prefer to consume it hot

RECIPES

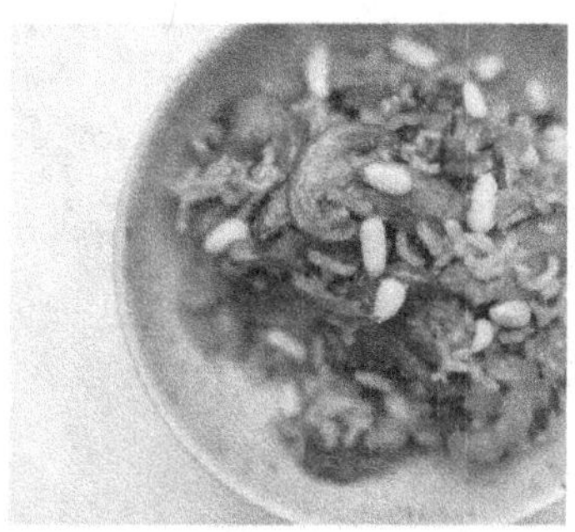

MUSHROOMS WITH
BROCCOLI

Ingredients

- 500 gr of broccoli
- 200 gr of mushrooms
- 2 tomatoes
- 1 dash of white wine
- oil, garlic and salt

Preparation

Crumble the broccoli into smaller florets, and cut the trunk into slices. In a saucepan with water, boil the broccoli until soft. then drain them and set aside.

While cooking the vegetables, wash and clean the mushrooms under running water and slice it. Then in a frying pan, brown the garlic with the mushrooms, tomatoes and broccoli. Add the vegetables and let it rest at the pan for a couple of minutes

Nutrition

ENJOY

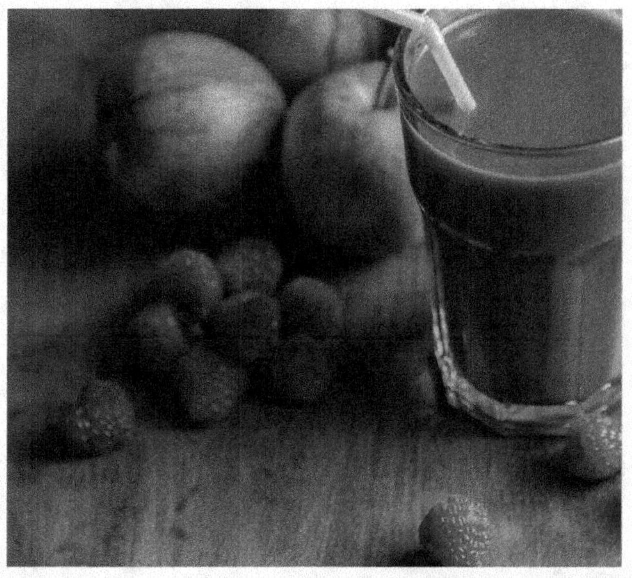

Charts
PLAN YOUR MEALS

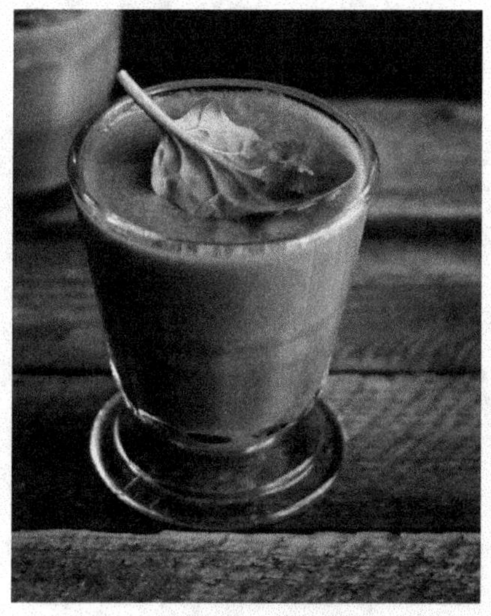

I INCLUDE HERE
SOME CHARTS

Take care of
your wellbeing

New Earth   @mariakrystalflames

Section 1

PLANNING YOUR MEALS

You can plan your meals for the next month or 3 months to help you with your groceries shopping list

30 DAYS ....

ACTION PLAN

- ○
- ○
- ○
- ○

60 DAYS ....

ACTION PLAN

- ○
- ○
- ○
- ○

90 DAYS ....

ACTION PLAN

- ○
- ○
- ○
- ○

Section 2

PLANNING AHEAD

A WEEKLY PLAN

Include here the recipes you like for a balanced week

Section 2

PLANNING AHEAD

A WEEKLY PLAN 2

Include here the recipes you like for a balanced week

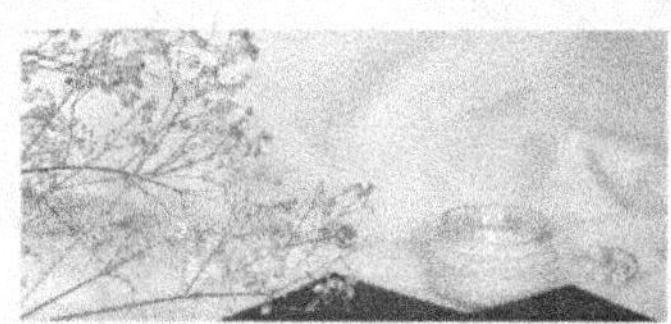

Section 3
ACTION STEPS

Choose the recipes that best serves your diet goals

1

2

3

notes

About
THE AUTHOR

María Casado Cuyás, born in Canary Islands, on July 25, when Syrius rises with the Sun, the day ¨Out of Time & Space¨ according to the Mayan Calendar, on Lion's Gate.

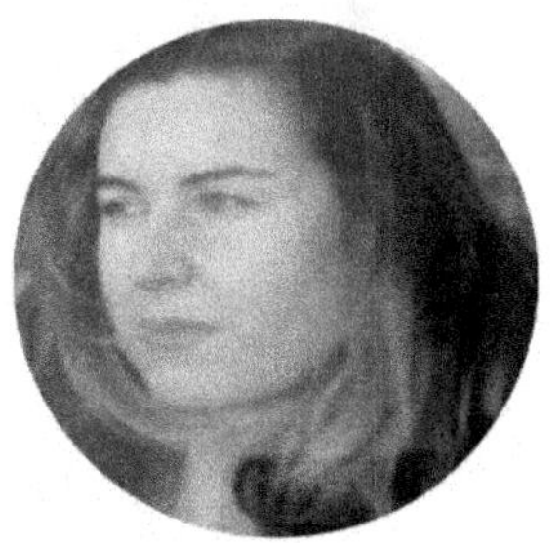

On that Zodiac Blueprint she has joined Heavens & Earth through her Art, in her paintings and books.

She has Lived in Paris to study Modern Anglosaxon Letters and French Literature.
Back to Spain, she founded the Communication Department with Press Media for Larousse Publishing House.
Her True Wish for All human beings is that her writings unfold the Inner Path Back Home to the Cosmic Ocean in Father's Heart

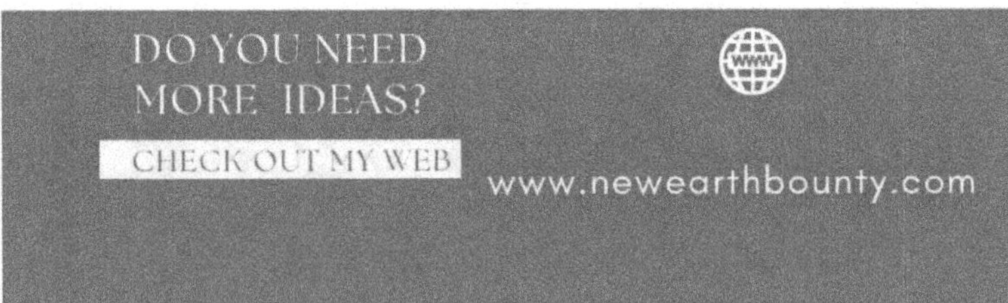